A Christian's Guide to Life
(Getting it Right)

– Elsie Oladimeji –

FASTPRINT PUBLISHING
PETERBOROUGH, ENGLAND

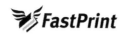

www.fast-print.net/store.php

A Christian's Guide to Life
Copyright © Elsie Oladimeji 2011

ISBN 978-184426-902-0

First published 2011 by
FASTPRINT PUBLISHING
Peterborough, England.

An environmentally friendly book printed and bound in England
by www.printondemand-worldwide.com

Mixed Sources
Product group from well-managed
forests, and other controlled sources
www.fsc.org Cert no. TT-COC-002641
© 1996 Forest Stewardship Council

FSC

PEFC Certified
This product is
from sustainably
managed forests
and controlled
sources
www.pefc.org

PEFC/16-33-415

This book is made entirely of chain-of-custody materials

Contents

Introduction

This book has been put together as an easy guide for Christians at all levels of growth, using Scripture to inform, equip and remind us of the basics of our Christianity which oftentimes we seem to forget or maybe do not even know. There is so much more to our faith than can be contained in a little book, but this one seeks to cover some key aspects. However, it is not exhaustive. It can be used as a tool for Home Groups, Bible Study, New Believers Classes or simply as a tool for spiritual growth - for the believer to be built up and to be better equipped to minister the dynamics of our faith to others in a simple but effective way.

It starts with, "Who is God?" so that anyone who picks this book up, who is searching for God may know who we know Him to be. The primary aim of this book is to stir the heart of the reader to seek after God, to lay hold of all that has been given to us through the death and resurrection of our Lord Jesus Christ, to live a victorious life here on earth en route to heaven, and to be a shining example of who a Christian should be.

Dedication

For the wonderful things You do, for calling me out of darkness into Your marvellous light, and for being the strength of my life, I dedicate this book to You - Father, Son and Holy Spirit. This book is for You, through You and about You - thank You.

1
Who Is God?

What can man possibly write about who God is that can adequately describe Him?

The easiest way to describe Him, is by allowing the scriptures to paint a picture of who He is in our hearts. What is certain though, is that He is not a figment of man's imagination nor is He so small that He can be limited to an image crafted by the hands of man. We do not use Scripture (the Bible) as "a way" to describe God, as if there are many other ways, but we use Scripture as "the way" to describe who He is and to test every other revelation that we may feel we have of Him. Having said this, even though we may get to know about Him through the Bible, we cannot really know Him except by His Spirit, as we accept Jesus Christ into our lives and spend quality time in fellowship with Him.

The first thing that we know about Him from Scripture (Genesis 1) is that He is the Creator of the heavens and the earth and all that is in them; but He is so much more than this and greatly desires that the people who He has made would come to know Him intimately.

There is a void in every man or woman that only God can fill. People may try to fill that void with other things - relationships, money, possessions, even so called "religion" but find that there is still some form of "emptiness" in them that nothing or no one else can fill, except the true and living God. He is standing at the door of every heart that has not received Him, and He is knocking - if you invite Him, He will come in and fill that void.

(If you have never invited Jesus Christ into your heart and would like to, please go to the last page of this book for Prayer of Salvation.)

Acts 17:22-31 NASB - Then Paul stood in the midst of the Areopagus and said, "Men of Athens, I perceive that in all things you are very religious; 23 for as I was passing through and considering the objects of your worship, I even found an altar with this inscription:

TO THE UNKNOWN GOD.

Therefore, the One whom you worship without knowing, Him I proclaim to you: 24 God, who made the world and everything in it, since He is Lord of heaven and earth, does not dwell in temples made with hands. 25 Nor is He worshiped with men's hands, as though He needed anything, since He gives to all life, breath, and all things. 26 And He has made from one blood every nation of men to dwell on all the face of the earth, and has determined their preappointed times and the boundaries of their dwellings, 27 so that they should seek the Lord, in the hope that they might grope for Him and find Him, though He is not far from each one of us; 28 for in Him we live and move and have our being, as also some of your own poets have said, 'For we are also

His offspring.' [29] *Therefore, since we are the offspring of God, we ought not to think that the Divine Nature is like gold or silver or stone, something shaped by art and man's devising.* [30] *Truly, these times of ignorance God overlooked, but now commands all men everywhere to repent,* [31] *because He has appointed a day on which He will judge the world in righteousness by the Man whom He has ordained. He has given assurance of this to all by raising Him from the dead.*

THE GODHEAD:

Through Scripture, particularly in the New Testament we learn of the unity of the Father, the Son and the Holy Spirit as three persons in one God. In Genesis 1:26 the Bible says: *"Then God said, "Let Us make man in our image"*, John 1:1-3 says this about the Lord Jesus: *"In the beginning was the Word, and the Word was with God, and the Word was God. He was in the beginning with God. All things were made through Him, and without Him nothing was made that was made."* Also John 14:8-11 says: *"Philip said to Him, "Lord, show us the Father, and it is sufficient for us."* [9] *Jesus said to him, "Have I been with you so long, and yet you have not known Me, Philip? He who has seen Me has seen the Father; so how can you say, 'Show us the Father'?* [10] *Do you not believe that I am in the Father, and the Father in Me? The words that I speak to you I do not speak on my own authority; but the Father who dwells in me does the works.* [11] *Believe Me that I am in the Father and the Father in Me, or else believe me for the sake of the works themselves."*

The Father sets the plan (Ephesians 1:3-5), the Son carries it out (John 1:1-5) and the Holy Spirit helps us individually to apply the plan to our lives (John 16:13).

The following are scriptures to help us grasp the distinct characteristics of God's Being:

THE FATHER

This depicts God's divine relationship with us, as not just God out there up in heaven, aloof from His people, but as a Father who loves us and has made a way for us to approach Him. The Father sets the "rules" for life, not to harm us but to do us good. It is impossible to have a relationship with the Father except through the Son (Jesus Christ) who paid the penalty for our sins so that we can have access to the throne of God.

Ephesians 1:3-5 NASB - Blessed be the God and Father of our Lord Jesus Christ, who has blessed us with every spiritual blessing in the heavenly places in Christ, ⁴ just as He chose us in Him before the foundation of the world, that we would be holy and blameless before Him in love ⁵ He predestined us to adoption as sons through Jesus Christ to Himself, according to the kind intention of His will,

Romans 8:15-16 - For you did not receive the spirit of bondage again to fear, but you received the Spirit of adoption by whom we cry out, "Abba, Father." ¹⁶ The Spirit Himself bears witness with our spirit that we are children of God,

THE SON

(Jesus Christ) - Our Lord and Saviour who came in the flesh as man to take upon Himself the punishment and death that was due to us for our transgressions, so that we may have access to all that is His. He gave His life and His blood on the Cross for the remission of sins, (past, present and future) and made as many as receive Him to become joint heirs with Him in the Kingdom of our God.

John 14:6 - Jesus said to him, "I am the way, the truth, and the life. No one comes to the Father except through Me.

Colossians 1:15-19 - He is the image of the invisible God, the firstborn over all creation. [16] For by Him all things were created that are in heaven and that are on earth, visible and invisible, whether thrones or dominions or principalities or powers. All things were created through Him and for Him. [17] And He is before all things, and in Him all things consist. [18] And He is the head of the body, the church, who is the beginning, the firstborn from the dead, that in all things He may have the preeminence. [19] For it pleased the Father that in Him all the fullness should dwell, [20] and by Him to reconcile all things to Himself, by Him, whether things on earth or things in heaven, having made peace through the blood of His cross.

For further reading:

John 1:1-5
Romans 5:12-21

THE HOLY SPIRIT

(Comforter, Helper, Advocate) - You cannot receive the Holy Spirit without first making Jesus Christ the Lord of your life. An unbeliever can be convicted by the Holy Spirit, but cannot have His indwelling Presence. He is the assurance of our salvation; as we receive Him and yield to Him, He will lead us into all truth and empower us to be who God had purposed us to be, to do all that we have to do, so that we can inherit all that Christ has for us.

John 14:16-17 - And I will pray the Father, and He will give you another Helper, that He may abide with you forever— [17] the Spirit of truth, whom the world cannot receive, because it neither sees Him nor knows Him; but you know Him, for He dwells with you and will be in you.

John 14:26 - But the Helper, the Holy Spirit, whom the Father will send in My name, He will teach you all things, and bring to your remembrance all things that I said to you.

Acts 1:8 - But you shall receive power when the Holy Spirit has come upon you; and you shall be witnesses to Me in Jerusalem, and in all Judea and Samaria, and to the end of the earth."

Having had a revelation of God, Job says in Job 42:5-6: *"I have heard of You by the hearing of the ear, but now my eye sees You. [6] Therefore I abhor myself, and repent in dust and ashes."* If you do not truly know God, you too can have a revelation of Him as you make Jesus Christ the Lord of your life and allow the Holy Spirit to reveal Him to your heart, through *the word (the Bible), through prayers, in worship and in any other way that He chooses to reveal Him to you.*

2
Who We Are In Christ

CHILDREN OF GOD

Not just His creation or children from a distance, but children who are intimate with Him who not only fellowship with Him, but who He talks to or desires to talk to in many ways too.

John 1:12 – But as many as received Him, to them He gave the right to become children of God, to those who believe in His name

Romans 8:14 – For as many as are led by the Spirit of God, these are sons of God.

Galatians 3:26 - For you are all sons of God through faith in Christ Jesus.

JOINT HEIRS WITH CHRIST

We have been given the right to partake in Christ's inheritance through our adoption as sons because of the work of redemption that Jesus accomplished for us on the Cross.

Romans 8:17 - And if children, then heirs—heirs of God and joint heirs with Christ, if indeed we suffer with Him, that we may also be glorified together.

Revelations 5:11-12 - Then I looked, and I heard the voice of many angels around the throne, the living creatures, and the elders; and the number of them was ten thousand times ten thousand, and thousands of thousands, [15] saying with a loud voice "Worthy is the Lamb who was Slain to receive power and riches and wisdom, and strength and honor and glory and blessing!"

For further reading:

Galatians 4:1-6

NEW MAN

Your old life up until the day you made Jesus Christ the Lord of your life is considered gone, you get a new start (You are born again!). It's like being given a clean slate to draw on and in His word He has given us what to draw with. Colossians 3:16 says: *"Let the word of Christ dwell in you richly in all wisdom..."*, so read the Bible and listen to the word of God being preached or taught and let your mind be renewed by it. In the scriptures, we get to know about the great power that has been made available to us; so that when the enemy (the devil) tries to come and draw his lies, his deceptions, his doubts, his fears, his distractions, his bitterness on the slate of our lives, we are better equipped to resist him.

2 Corinthians 5:17 - Therefore, if anyone is in Christ, he is a new creation; old things have passed away; behold, all things have become new.

Galatians 2:20 - I have been crucified with Christ; it is no longer I who live, but Christ lives in me; and the life which I now live in the flesh I live by faith in the Son of God, who loved me and gave Himself for me.

THE RIGHTEOUSNESS OF GOD

Our right standing with God is not because of our good works or our righteous acts, it is simply a free gift from God, therefore the enemy should not be able to condemn us if we know our rights. If it were by works, then we'll have to be perfect, because that is what God expects, but because He knows that we will always fall short of His standard for perfection, He gave us Christ and inputted His (Christ's) righteousness to us.

Nevertheless, He expects us to be righteous (to obey His commandments which are not burdensome, but have been given for our own good); it is part of the package, so that we may live a fruitful life here on earth and leave no room for the adversary to oppress us by continuing in sin. We should not sin; as children of God, sin should be strange and uncomfortable for us, however if we do sin we have an advocate with the Father, Jesus Christ *"In Him we have redemption through His blood, the forgiveness of sins, according to the riches of His grace"* (Ephesians 1:7).

The parable of the prodigal son (Luke 15:11 -32), typifies the mercy of the Father. If you are a prodigal son (one who has strayed from the Lord), return to the Father now, He is waiting for you with open arms, if you are not a prodigal son, thank God! May you never stray from His grace, because no one knows the day or the hour of Christ's return, neither do we know the day or the time that our journey here on earth will end. So do not get caught outside of Christ!

2 Corinthians 5:21 - For He made Him who knew no sin to be sin for us, that we might become the righteousness of God in Him.

Ephesians 2:8-9 - For by grace you have been saved through faith, and that not of yourselves; it is the gift of God, [9] not of works, lest anyone should boast. [10] For we are His workmanship, created in Christ Jesus for good works, which God prepared beforehand that we should walk in them.

For further reading:

Romans 5:6-19

CITIZENS OF HEAVEN

In all that we do we must remember that we are sojourners and pilgrims on this earth, and what matters most is our eternal destination. We should fix our eyes on things above and not on earthly things. As it is written in 1 Timothy 6:7: "... we brought nothing into this world, and it is certain we shall carry nothing out."

John 17:14-16 - I have given them Your word; and the world has hated them because they are not of the world, just as I am not of the world. I do not pray that You should take them out of the world, but that You should keep them from the evil one. They are not of the world, just as I am not of the world.

1 Peter 2:11-12 NLT - Dear friends, I warn you as "temporary residents and foreigners" to keep away from worldly desires that wage war against your very souls. 12 Be careful to live properly among your unbelieving neighbors. Then even if they accuse you of doing wrong, they will see your honorable behavior, and they will give honor to God when he judges the world.

For further reading:

Colossians 3:1-4
Matthew 6:19-21
Mark 8:36-38

SPIRITUAL PEOPLE

We are not mere men and as such should not be led by the flesh whose works manifest as these: adultery, fornication, uncleanness, wantonness, idol worship, witchcraft, hatred, being quarrelsome, jealousies, wrath, selfish ambitions, envy, murders, drunkenness revelries and other things like these; but instead we should allow the Holy Spirit to lead us in righteousness and in power (Galatians 5:16-18).

1 Corinthians 3:3 - for you are still carnal. For where there are envy, strife, and divisions among you, are you not carnal and behaving like mere men?

Galatians 5:22-25 NIV - But the fruit of the Spirit is love, joy, peace, patience, kindness, goodness, faithfulness, [23]gentleness and self-control. Against such things there is no law.[24]Those who belong to Christ Jesus have crucified the sinful nature with its passions and desires. [25] Since we live by the Spirit, let us keep in step with the Spirit.

For further reading:

Galatians 5:16-26

AMBASSADORS OF CHRIST

As Ambassadors of Christ, we must do our best to let the difference show in our words and by our actions. Our job description is to spread the good news of Christ to all men and to demonstrate His compassion, so that the world can be reconciled back to God. He has given us our commission in Mark 16:15-20, which is to preach the gospel to the world - with signs and wonders following. Note here that as believers in Christ, and therefore His ambassadors, we are not to chase after signs and wonders, but rather they are supposed to follow us. He endues us with power from above as the Holy Spirit comes upon us (Acts 1:8), and the Holy Spirit equips us with the necessary gift or gifts (1 Corinthians 12:4-11) that we need to function in the various roles that He assigns to us.

2 Corinthians 5:19-20 - That is, that God was in Christ reconciling the world to Himself, not imputing their trespasses to them, and has committed to us the word of reconciliation. ²⁰ Now then, we are ambassadors for Christ, as though God were pleading through us: we implore you on Christ's behalf, be reconciled to God.

SALT OF THE EARTH

Salt is an essential ingredient with over a hundred uses. Imagine salt losing its flavour, it's like having so much potential, but being ineffective! That's how we are as Christians, "ineffective" if we sit back and do nothing with the great potential that God has put in us to make a difference here on earth for Him.

Matthew 5:13 – You are the salt of the earth; but if the salt loses its flavor, how shall it be seasoned? It is then good for nothing but to be thrown out and trampled underfoot by men.

LIGHT OF THE WORLD

As light chases away darkness, so we are to light up the places that God sends us to and cause the radiance of Christ's glory in us to dispel whatever darkness that might be there.

Matthew 5:14-16 - You are the light of the world. A city that is set on a hill cannot be hidden. [15] Nor do they light a lamp and put it under a basket, but on a lampstand, and it gives light to all who are in the house. [16] Let your light so shine before men, that they may see your good works and glorify your Father in heaven.

A DWELLING PLACE FOR GOD

The Lord needs us to do His work here on earth, because He has created the earth for humans to rule in. Though God can move in His sovereignty, He does not always do this without our cooperation if it will break His word; this is the faithfulness of God, that we can trust that His word is infallible. What a better world this would be if the Lord had more dwelling places! This is why we must spread the good news of Christ so that the Kingdom of God may flourish and souls may be delivered from Satan's grip and come to know the truth.

Through His Spirit in us, He stirs us up, He equips us, He empowers us and works His purposes through us if we let Him. He will not use us against our will. God needs us to pray, to speak the right things and to do the right things, so that He can act. Jesus Christ being our example; came to earth as man and was empowered by the Holy Spirit - He prayed, spoke the mind of God and did the will of God, and has also given us this pattern to follow. 2 Corinthians 2:14 reads: *"Now thanks be to God who always leads us in triumph in Christ, and through us diffuses the fragrance of His knowledge in every place."*

Ephesians 2:22 - in whom you also are being built together for a dwelling place of God in the Spirit

1 Corinthians 6:19 - Or do you not know that your body is the temple of the Holy Spirit who is in you, whom you have from God, and you are not your own?

MORE THAN CONQUERORS

As more than conquerors we are to rise above whatever circumstances we face. Jesus says in John 16:33: *"These things I have spoken to you, that in Me you may have peace. In the world you will have tribulation; but be of good cheer, I have overcome the world."* The truth of the matter is that the devil's fight is not only against Christians, but also against all mankind. However, those who are not in Christ are easy prey, because the devil knows that God loves them but because they are not laying hold of all that God has for them, he lulls them into a false sense of security and by the time that they know that things are not quite right, it may be too late for some. 2 Corinthians 4:3-4 says: *"But even if our gospel is veiled, it is veiled to those who are perishing, whose minds the god of this age has blinded, who do not believe, lest the light of the gospel of the glory of Christ, who is the image of God, should shine on them"*

Our fight is not in our own strength, it is simply by the word of God and from the position of authority in Christ – the outcome is already settled, we are triumphant! Jesus says in Luke 10:19: "Behold, I give you the authority to trample on serpents and scorpions, and over all the power of the enemy, and nothing shall by any means hurt you". What we can change we change, through prayer and taking the necessary actions; but what we cannot change, His grace has been made available for us to bear it.

We have to change our mindset and renew our minds in line with who God says we are in Christ. He wants us to "rise up and shine", so that His glory may be revealed through us to a dying world. We are not to live defeated lives as though we have no hope, but rather we are to stand firm in Him and upon His word and we will walk in victory.

Romans 8:35-37 - Who shall separate us from the love of Christ? Shall tribulation, or distress, or persecution, or famine, or nakedness, or peril, or sword? As it is written: "For Your sake we are killed all day long; we are accounted as sheep for the slaughter." Yet in all these things we are more than conquerors through Him who loved us

---

For further reading:
Romans 5:3-5
Philippians 4:13
Ephesians 6:10-18

MADE TO RULE

We are special, royalty, chosen ones; we are made in His image, after His likeness, set apart for the Master's use. We can move "mountains" through prayer and change situations, because we have been given the authority to do so. Jesus Christ says in Matthew 16:19 (NASB): *"I will give you the keys of the kingdom of heaven; and whatever you bind on earth shall have been bound in heaven, and whatever you loose on earth shall have been loosed in heaven."* Our prayer is: "May Your Kingdom come, O Lord and Your will be done on earth as it is in heaven" - after the manner that Jesus Christ taught the disciples in Matthew Chapter six verse ten.

1 Peter 2:9-10 - But you are a chosen generation, a royal priesthood, a holy nation, His own special people, that you may proclaim the praises of Him who called you out of darkness into His marvellous light; who once were not a people but are now the people of God, who had not obtained mercy but now have obtained mercy.

Revelations 1:6 - and has made us kings and priests to His God and Father, to Him be glory and dominion forever and ever. Amen.

2 Corinthians 10:3-6 - For though we walk in the flesh, we do not war according to the flesh. For the weapons of our warfare are not carnal but mighty in God for pulling down strongholds, casting down arguments and every high thing that exalts itself against the knowledge of God, bringing every thought into captivity to the obedience of Christ, and being ready to punish all disobedience when your obedience is fulfilled.

For further reading:
Genesis 1:26-28
Matthew 18:18

3
What Is Ours

The first thing that we have in Jesus Christ is forgiveness of sin, which is the basis of all that we have received in Him. He paid the penalty for our sins on the cross and set us free from the evil consequences that would have been due to us, so that God's blessings can reach us. In Colossians 1:13-14, it says that: *"He has delivered us from the power of darkness and conveyed us into the kingdom of the Son of His love, in whom we have redemption through His blood, the forgiveness of sins."*

Jesus did not go to the cross to give us an ordinary life. Salvation is a total package – it starts from when we give our lives to Christ, but does not end there. Jesus likens Himself to the good Shepherd, and definitely a good Shepherd's sheep is not raggedly. John 10:10-11 says: *"The thief does not come except to steal, and to kill, and to destroy. I have come that they may have life, and that they may have it more abundantly. I am the good shepherd. The good shepherd gives His life for the sheep."*

As joint heirs with Christ, we are also partakers of His kingdom inheritance. Revelations 5:11-12 details Christ's inheritance, which we are also entitled to share in, not only in eternity with Him, but also here on earth. They are as follows:

POWER

Acts 1:8 - *But you shall receive power when the Holy Spirit has come upon you; and you shall be witnesses to Me in Jerusalem, and in all Judea and Samaria, and to the end of the earth.*

Power here is from the Greek word "dunamis" which relates to miraculous power. Through the baptism of the Holy Spirit we have been endued with power from above, with the main purpose of testifying of the Lordship of Jesus Christ and demonstrating His compassion and mercy. With this also, we have been giving the authority to destroy the works of the devil as we stand in faith proclaiming the word of the Lord with power (Luke 10:19).

> *For further reading:*
> Matthew 18:18
> Matthew 16:19
> John 14:12

RICHES

2 Corinthians 8:9 NIV - For you know the grace of our Lord Jesus Christ, that though he was rich, yet for your sakes he became poor, so that you through his poverty might become rich.

To put a caution here, this is not talking about covetousness or greed - we are not to fight and war or compromise to be rich, but riches that are acquired through the blessings and favour of God. This is so that we are not only blessed ourselves, but are a blessing to others. The balance in scripture is found in 1 Timothy 6:6-10 NLT – *"Yet true godliness with contentment is itself great wealth. After all, we brought nothing with us when we came into the world, and we can't take anything with us when we leave it. So if we have enough food and clothing, let us be content. But people who long to be rich fall into temptation and are trapped by many foolish and harmful desires that plunge them into ruin and destruction. For the love of money is the root of all kinds of evil. And some people, craving money, have wandered from the true faith and pierced themselves with many sorrows."*

God wants us to be rich, but He does not want us to be consumed by it. Psalm 62:10 warns us not to get carried away even if riches increase, because we know that as Matthew 6:21 says *"For where your treasure is, there your heart will be also."* Money in itself is neither good nor bad, but we must not be overcome by the love of it, instead whatever we have should be acquired in a way and used in a way that does not bring reproach, but rather brings glory to God.

Riches here, is not just talking about money. Jesus Christ deprived himself and forsook the shame so that we might have a richly fulfilled life here on earth and also a glorious eternity with Him when our time here on earth is over.

WISDOM

James 1:5 NIV - If any of you lacks wisdom, he should ask God, who gives generously to all without finding fault, and it will be given to him.

Not earthly wisdom, but godly wisdom. *"But the wisdom that is from above is first pure, then peaceable, gentle, willing to yield, full of mercy and good fruits, without partiality and without hypocrisy." (James 3:17)*

STRENGTH

2 Corinthians 12:9 - And He said to me, "My grace is sufficient for you, for My strength is made perfect in weakness." Therefore most gladly I will rather boast in my infirmities, that the power of Christ may rest upon me.

The first and main area of our life that we need His strength in is in our inner man, because if we are strong there, then we are better able to overcome in whatever situation we find ourselves, and not allow the circumstances of life to overwhelm us. This is Paul's prayer in Ephesians 3:16: *"that He would grant you, according to the riches of His glory, to be strengthened with might through His Spirit in the inner man"* (Make this your prayer too!)

Strength also includes, divine health: physically, mentally and emotionally. As written in 1 Peter 2:24 (NASB): *"He himself bore our sins in his body on the tree, so that we might die to sins and live for righteousness; by his wounds you have been healed."*

HONOUR

John 12:26 NIV - Whoever serves me must follow me; and where I am, my servant also will be. My Father will honor the one who serves me.

When God created mankind He crowned us with glory and honour (Psalm 8:5), but man through sin allowed himself to be clothed with shame and dishonour instead. Thank God that in Christ Jesus this shame is taken away and our glory and honour are restored. What an honour for us to be called children of God, not just children but sons. Sons, because in those days, sons were esteemed higher than daughters and had first and greater claim to inheritance, in some cases total claim; unfortunately this is still the practice in some cultures. However, in Christ as concerns our inheritance, we are all termed sons; for there is neither Jew nor Greek, slave nor free, male nor female in Him, we are all one in Him – no one is inferior (Galatians 3:26-29). This is the Lord's way of saying to us that we are not just children, but highly esteemed children who are entitled to an inheritance in Christ.

GLORY

2 Corinthians 3:14-18 NASB - But their minds were hardened; for until this very day at the reading of the old covenant the same veil remains unlifted, because it is removed in Christ. [15]But to this day whenever Moses is read, a veil lies over their heart; *16but whenever a person turns to the Lord, the veil is taken away. 17Now the Lord is the Spirit, and where the Spirit of the Lord is, there is liberty. 18But we all, with unveiled face, beholding as in a mirror the glory of the Lord, are being transformed into the same image from glory to glory, just as from the Lord, the Spirit.*

BLESSING

Ephesians 1:3 - *Blessed be the God and Father of our Lord Jesus Christ, who has blessed us with every spiritual blessing in the heavenly places in Christ*

God has blessed us with everything that is beneficial to us so that we may have a fruitful life here on earth and sweet life forevermore with Him in eternity. He became a curse for us (Galatians 3:7-14), so that we can be free to inherit the blessings that He promised to Abraham and his sons through faith.

All these have been made available to us in Jesus Christ, but we must lay hold of them by faith.

4
What Is Expected Of Us

1. That we love God with all our heart, with all our soul and with all our strength (Deuteronomy 6:5) - A way to prove your love for God is by doing His will and keeping His commandments.

John 14:21 - He who has My commandments and keeps them, it is he who loves Me. And he who loves Me will be loved by My Father, and I will love him and manifest Myself to him.

2. That we put God first in all things - Let doing His will be our primary focus.

Matthew 6:33 - But seek first the kingdom of God and His righteousness, and all these things shall be added to you.

3. Be Water Baptised (Mark 16:16) - this is the public affirmation of our commitment to Christ. It is not an

option, but a command from the Lord to all those who believe in Him. It symbolises our being buried with Him (death to the old life) and as He rose up from the dead, even so we should also rise up and walk in the new life that we have in Him.

Romans 6:4 - Therefore we were buried with Him through baptism into death, that just as Christ was raised from the dead by the glory of the Father, even so we also should walk in newness of life.

4. That we live our lives in a manner worthy of those professing to be God's (Colossians 1:9-11; Colossians 3:1-10) - As the saying goes, "Actions speak louder than words", therefore we must let our Christianity be evident by the way we live our lives.

Ephesians 4:17-24 - This I say, therefore, and testify in the Lord, that you should no longer walk as the rest of the Gentiles walk, in the futility of their mind, having their understanding darkened, being alienated from the life of God, because of the ignorance that is in them, because of the blindness of their heart; who, being past feeling, have given themselves over to lewdness, to work all uncleanness with greediness. But you have not so learned Christ, if indeed you have heard Him and have been taught by Him, as the truth is in Jesus: that you put off, concerning your former conduct, the old man which grows corrupt according to the deceitful lusts, and be renewed in the spirit of your mind, and that you put on the new man which was created according to God, in true righteousness and holiness.

5. Present our bodies as living sacrifices, holy and acceptable to Him (Romans 12:1) - It is our

responsibility to set godly standards for the world to follow rather than follow trends and patterns set out by the world that do not glorify God.

1 Corinthians 6:19-20 - Or do you not know that your body is the temple of the Holy Spirit who is in you, whom you have from God, and you are not your own? ²⁰ for you were bought at a price; therefore glorify God in your body and in your spirit, which are God's.

6. Love one another (John 15:12; Romans 12:10; 1 Corinthians 13) - God is Love, therefore if we are His, we must love one another - as hard as it may seem at times, it really is possible! If we do not have Christ it would have been impossible, but thank God that we do. Therefore, because we do, we have the Holy Spirit our Helper to help us love even the seemingly unlovable.

Matthew 22:28-29 - Jesus said to him, " 'You shall love the LORD your God with all your heart, with all your soul, and with all your mind.' ³⁸ This is the first and great commandment. ³⁹ And the second is like it: 'You shall love your neighbour as yourself.'

This is the grace of God - that God demonstrated His love for us by dying for us while we were still sinners (Romans 5:8). He didn't wait for us to repent or to change, but He purchased the forgiveness for our sins by making atonement with His own blood on the Cross and wants us to forgive others too when they err against us, whether they deserve it or not. He uses the parable of the unforgiving servant in Matthew Chapter eighteen verses twenty one to thirty five to minister His desire to us. Also

Matthew 6:14-15 says: *"For if you forgive men when they sin against you, your heavenly Father will also forgive you. ¹⁵But if you do not forgive men their sins, your Father will not forgive your sins."*

7. Declare the Good News of Christ to others - it is our duty to let those around us know who we are and what we believe and why we believe what we believe (share your own experience of Christ with them) and tell them about the love of God for them, manifested through the sacrifice of Christ on the Cross; so that they too may have eternal life, and enjoy the goodness of God that we enjoy or should enjoy.

Mark 16:15-18 - And He said to them, "Go into all the world and preach the gospel to every creature. He who believes and is baptized will be saved; but he who does not believe will be condemned. And these signs will follow those who believe: In My name they will cast out demons; they will speak with new tongues; they will take up serpents; and if they drink anything deadly, it will by no means hurt them; they will lay hands on the sick, and they will recover.

5
How Do We Get It Right?

1. Spend quality time in God's presence

Psalm 16:11 – You will show me the path of life; In Your presence is fullness of joy; at Your right hand are pleasures forevermore.

> ➤ Praise and Worship the Lord with your words and with songs.
> ➤ Pray (In the Spirit and in your understanding)
> ➤ Take time to be quiet before Him and allow Him to minister to your heart
> ➤ Fast regularly

As we spend quality time in God's presence, we get to know Him more, we get to love Him more and we are filled more and more with His Spirit. The Holy Spirit is the One who helps us to change, but we have to be willing and desirous of change. To be filled with the Spirit is not a once and for all experience, we need to be filled daily as we allow Him to lead us by spending quality time in fellowship with Him.

As you build up your spirit man (the inner man) in the Lord, you will have strength not only to resist the temptations of the flesh, but also to triumph over them. It says in Jude 1:20: *"But you, beloved, building yourselves up on your most holy faith, praying in the Holy Spirit"*

2. Read the Bible

Colossians 3:16 - Let the word of Christ dwell in you richly in all wisdom, teaching and admonishing one another in psalms and hymns and spiritual songs, singing with grace in your hearts to the Lord.

Study it, meditate on it, and apply it to your daily life - be a doer of the word, not just one who hears and does not do what he ought to do with what he hears (James 1:22). Prayer without the word or the word without prayer is like a car without fuel. Do not simply wait till the word is preached to you; get into the word yourself and see if what is preached to you tallies with God's word. The Bible tells us to test every spirit if they are of God (1 John 4:1), but how do we do this if we do not know what the word of God says?

3. Be planted in a Church

Hebrews 10:25 - not forsaking the assembling of ourselves together, as is the manner of some, but exhorting one another, and so much the more as you see the Day approaching.

Psalm 92:13 - Those who are planted in the house of the LORD shall flourish in the courts of our God.

Do not only read the word, but also be part of a church where you will hear the undiluted word of God preached and taught. Be in a church where you can grow and fellowship with other believers and be equipped to serve God. Collectively, we are the body of Christ; the arm cannot function alone without the shoulder, neither can the shoulder function alone without the chest, it must be knit together as a body and the body knit to the Head, who is Christ. You cannot be a "lone ranger" Christian, you need other Christians around you, so you can grow together and also when you are weak they can encourage you, stand with you and pray with you (vice versa); and bring correction (in love) if need be.

4. Have faith in God

Hebrews 11:6 - But without faith it is impossible to please Him, for he who comes to God must believe that He is, and that He is a rewarder of those who diligently seek Him.

The Lord has provided a lot for us through the Cross other than the remission of sins, but we have to *"fight the good fight of faith"* (1 Timothy 6:12) to lay hold of all that He has already released to us. You cannot simply fold your arms, wait and do nothing, for *"faith without works is dead"* (James 2:20). Though we may go through various trials, some because of the choices and decisions that we make, we remain confident in the fact that God loves us and that as we reach out to Him, He will work everything out for our good.

It is our responsibility to resist the devil when he comes with his temptations, by declaring what the Word of God says concerning the situation. We have our example in Matthew Chapter four, when Jesus was tempted by the devil in the wilderness; Jesus overcame him by the word of God. God always backs us up, however we have to do the resisting, because He has already given us the victory over all the works of the devil. So just stand your ground and declare the victory that you have through the blood of Jesus. The key to our victory is in His word – SUBMIT to God, RESIST the devil and he will flee from you (James 4:7).

5. Sow good seeds

Galatians 6:7 - Do not be deceived, God is not mocked; for whatever a man sows, that he will also reap.

Luke 6:38 - Give, and it will be given to you: good measure, pressed down, shaken together, and running over will be put into your bosom. For with the same measure that you use, it will be measured back to you."

Malachi 3:10 NIV - Bring the whole tithe into the storehouse, that there may be food in my house. Test me in this," says the LORD Almighty, *"and see if I will not throw open the floodgates of heaven and pour out so much blessing that you will not have room enough for it.*

One principle that is certain on earth, whether you are a believer or not, is found in Genesis 8:22: *"While the earth remains, seedtime and harvest, cold and heat, winter and summer, and day and night shall not cease."* In order words, what you sow, you will reap and not just the same amount – you reap much more! Therefore, whatever you would like others to do to you, do also to them (Matthew 7:12). Give of your resources: time, money, whatever is needed or the best you are able to give in furtherance of God's work and you shall surely be rewarded with much more (our primary reason for giving though should not be for the reward, but for the love of God and the love of others).

6. Keep good company

1 Corinthians 15:33 NIV - Do not be misled: "Bad company corrupts good character."

There is an adage that says: *"show me your friends and I'll tell you who you are"*. Friends that you are not able to influence for good may end up influencing you negatively. Even though you may not necessarily stop talking with them or being friendly, you must not always be found "hanging around" with those who are living their lives contrary to what you believe; get hooked up instead with those who believe what you believe and who will encourage you in your walk with the Lord.

For further reading:
2 Corinthians 6:14-17

---

7. Guard your heart diligently

Proverbs 4:23 - Keep your heart with all diligence, for out of it spring the issues of life.

Be careful what you entertain in your heart, stay away from things that may contaminate your thinking - the more you meditate on evil, you will be overcome by it. Use the list in Philippians 4:8 as a guideline: *"... whatever things are true, whatever things are noble, whatever things are just, whatever things are pure, whatever things are lovely, whatever things are of good report, if there is any virtue and if there is anything praiseworthy—meditate on these things."*

Finally, we must recognise that we are who we are because of God's grace and mercy, and all our attempts to live right would be in vain without Him. We are however enjoined by Jesus to "carry our cross daily and follow Him" (Luke 9:23).

"The Cross" is a place of sacrifice; this means that we have to sacrifice our desires and aspirations when they conflict with His word and His will for our lives, knowing that His thoughts and plans for us are good ones. There is coming a day when the trumpet will sound, and the Lord will return for His Church, no one knows what day or time this would be, but it shall surely happen as written (1 Thessalonians 4:13-18; Matthew 24:29-31). Even if He delays because of His loving kindness not desiring that any should perish (2 Peter 3:9), there is still an appointed time that we must all put off our earthly flesh and leave this world - whichever comes first, we know that we have a home with Him if we continue in the faith. Knowing this, what manner of people should we be in conduct?

Jesus says in John 15:5-8: *"I am the vine, you are the branches. He who abides in Me, and I in him, bears much fruit; for without Me you can do nothing. [6] If anyone does not abide in Me, he is cast out as a branch and is withered; and they gather them and throw them into the fire, and they are burned. [7] If you abide in Me, and My words abide in you, you will ask what you desire, and it shall be done for you. [8] By this My Father is glorified, that you bear much fruit; so you will be My disciples."*
If you have truly come to know the Lord, you will no doubt realise that there is no greater joy here on earth than that which you find in relationship with Him, and there is no true peace without Him. His commandments are in no way burdensome and anything He will have you do, though at times sacrificial, is not unbearable because He makes His grace available to you as you need it.

Enjoy your walk with Him and remember to be a WITNESS for Christ!

SOME USEFUL PRAYERS FROM SCRIPTURE

Lord,

- Work in me both to will and to act in a manner that pleases you. (Philippians 2:13)
- Let the words of my mouth and the meditation of my heart be pleasing to You. (Psalm 19:14)
- Show me Your ways and teach me how to walk in them. (Psalm 25:4)
- Lead me in Your truth and teach me. (Psalm 25:5)
- Order my steps. (Psalm 37:23)
- May I walk worthy of You, fully pleasing You in all things. (Colossians 1:10)
- Grant me wisdom and revelation that I may know You more. (Ephesians 1:17)
- Let me understand what it is that you are calling me to do. (Ephesians 1:18)
- Strengthen me by Your spirit with power in my inward man. (Ephesians 3:15)
- Fill me with Your fullness. (Ephesians 3:19)

- May your word dwell richly in me. (Colossians 3:16)
- Fill me with the knowledge of Your will with wisdom and spiritual understanding. (Colossians 1:9)

PRAYER OF SALVATION

That if you confess with your mouth, "Jesus is Lord," and believe in your heart that God raised him from the dead, you will be saved. For it is with your heart that you believe and are justified, and it is with your mouth that you confess and are saved. As the Scripture says, "Anyone who trusts in him will never be put to shame." (Romans 10:9-11 NIV)

Pray this simple prayer:

Jesus Christ, I invite you into my heart and into my life to be my Lord and my Saviour. Please forgive me my sins and cleanse me from all unrighteousness. I repent of my sins and renounce them all. I believe that by faith I am now saved and born again and any claim of Satan over my life has been broken by your sacrifice on the cross. I receive your Holy Spirit into my heart.

I thank you Lord because according to your word in 2 Corinthians 5:17, old things have passed away and all things have become new for me today in your name.

Amen

If you have said this prayer, please find a Bible-believing, Spirit-filled Church to go to and tell as many people as you can about your new life. I pray that you will be blessed and filled with the knowledge of God.

Other titles by this Author:

Into the Master's Hand *(Journal of a Christian)*